Why Am I Eating This?

Is this the nourishment I need?

2ND EDITION

7 SIMPLE STEPS TO RE-TRAIN

YOUR MIND ABOUT FOOD

Sandy Robertson, RN, MSN, CHTP, CMIP

Illustrations by Gabrielle Balsz

WHY AM I EATING THIS?

7 SIMPLE STEPS TO RE-TRAIN

YOU MIND ABOUT FOOD

Sandy Robertson,RN, MSN, CHTP, CMIP

Illustrations by Gabrielle Balsz.

ISBN: 979-8-85775-271-5

"With love and gratitude to:
Mom who taught me how to celebrate and appreciate good food
and Dad, who taught me it was ok to say "no thank you, I'm full.""

CONTENTS

Chapter Three

Chapter Four

Chapter Five

Chapter Six

Chapter Seven

Chapter Eight

CHAPTER ONE

HEART OF THE MATTER: SELF AWARENESS AND MINDFULNESS

Step 1: Self Awareness

- Why do I overeat when I don't need food?
- What's in it for me?
- Why, when I know what I should eat, do I keep eating what I shouldn't?
- Am I bored, annoyed, distressed, or just lazy?
- What emotion am I stuffing instead of expressing?

Why Am I Eating This? is a little book with a big message. It puts a spotlight on the link between self-awareness and what and when we eat. Through a series of easy yet revealing exercises that pose probing questions to guide you toward self-discovery, you will unearth your "eating blueprint:" what governs you to eat, why, how much and when. Your eating blueprint is your conditioned response to food; it's the reason you default to automatic pilot when you're around food. At the end of the book, you will get to re-design it; to create a blueprint that is just for you.

The obesity statistics are alarming.

Approximately 35% of adult Americans over the age of 20 are obese, according to the Centers for Disease Control and Prevention. (www.cdc.gov/2008) These numbers remind us that millions of people don't know how, when, or why to stop eating too much—no matter how many diet books they read. Some of their eating habits are deeply rooted, with causes that have nothing to do with nutrition or levels of physical hunger.

Why do people keep eating when they know they should stop? Why Am I Eating This? will explore some of the answers and demonstrate how to eat in a more conscious way. It gets to the heart of the matter by helping you get underneath your default overeating patterns when you go on "automatic pilot" and can't seem to stop. The magical keys are self-awareness and mindfulness, moment to moment.

Self Awareness

I decided to write this book after counseling hundreds of individual clients over the years who boiled their eating problems down to one thing: they had no clue how much they were really eating and realized that quite often they were eating when they weren't even hungry.

In fact, I have heard people say "Why did I eat that" or "Why did I just stuff myself?" I even heard someone say it out loud at Christmas dinner once, after stuffing themselves without pausing to stop: "Why am I still eating?" I hear multiple variations of these words but they all cover the same theme: why do I put food in my mouth when I'm not even hungry?

Here are some examples of what my clients have discovered, after taking the time to tune in to what was really going on:

- As a busy sales executive, traveling almost nonstop, Robin noticed she was piling on the pounds, eating on an expense account. Client breakfasts and snacks reminded Robin of how her grandmother offered her snacks when she got home from school to welcome and comfort her. She realized she was overeating to give herself comfort. Once she started keeping a food log, it became apparent to her when and where all of her excess calories were coming from, and when; snacking in the car, late in the afternoon and she could be more deliberate about cutting down.

- When she was a child, Jane was told to eat everything on her plate because it was the polite thing to do. Now all grown up, she finds herself cleaning her plate wherever she goes. She realized she was overeating out of habit, with voices from long ago still in her mind. When she started rating her fullness and hunger, she discovered that she kept on eating way past the point where she was full, out of habit.

- Every time a client doesn't live up to his expectations, Doug indulges in an evening of pizza and submarine sandwiches. He figures he's entitled to this reward for all the hard work he put forth. It reminds him of how his mother would reward him with food, especially when things didn't go his way. When Doug combined keeping a food log with rating his hunger, he realized

- he was consuming a ridiculous amount of food. Most

  of all, he realized he was feeding his emotions, not because he needed the fuel for his body's health.

- After a difficult day at work, Julie treats herself to a king-size bag of chips with cheese dip. She figures she deserves this for putting up with all the stress, for going to a job she really doesn't like, and for being underappreciated and underpaid. When it was pointed out to Julie that keeping a food log combined with using breathing and relaxation exercises could work better for her as a stress management technique, she easily lost weight. She started nourishing her soul instead of her cravings.

- Jackie realized she was eating to spite her mother. Her mother wanted her to be thin and the two were often at war over her weight. Eating was an easy way to get back at her mother in a passive way. It was her way of saying, "Ha, ha. You want me to be thin, I'll show you." Jackie went to a two-day meditation retreat and realized the only one she was spiting was herself. She started exercising more and using mindfulness meditation techniques and she no longer feels the need to get back at her mother.

These are all examples of people turning to food on impulse, without paying attention or feeling the real source of their discomfort: themselves. If they could just tune in, pause to delay the impulse, and instead choose a healthier, more productive action in that moment they would feel more empowered and less in need of stuffing their feelings. "Stuffing feelings" is the way in which people avoid feeling or expressing their emotions by submerging and numbing them through eating. But as we all know, that is a temporary fix.

This book will give you a map to navigate away from self-sabotaging patterns and your "automatic pilot" relationship with food. In its place will be a new self-nurturing, healthy and empowering connection with food as fuel. I often tell students in my workshops that they are going to learn how to change their approach to food. It is not meant to replace therapy by a qualified medical professional who can help you delve into your own patterns in more detail. But *Why Am I Eating This?* may just be the key that unlocks the door to permanent weight loss for you.

Why This Book Is Different from Other Diet Books

Despite the astonishing amount of information and discussions about weight loss, few diet books address the core of the problem. Diet books tell you what you already know—eat less and exercise more. This book does not contain lists of foods to eat and foods to avoid; there are no menu plans, no charts with lists of caloric or fat content. Instead of recommending what to eat and what not to eat, I am inviting you to pay attention to **what**, **when** and **why** you are eating.

I also recommend getting regular exercise, at least 30 minutes a day, providing your doctor has no objection. Exercise not only burns calories, it helps your body to work more efficiently, and it creates muscle, which burns calories at a faster rate. Exercise helps keep your cardiovascular system working efficiently, your heart pumping the way it was meant to pump. It also gets oxygen flowing to your brain, causing you to feel more awake and energized. And for some people, endorphins being released by their brain when they exercise gives them what is known as a "natural high." It is an overall great way to reduce stress, enjoy leisure activity, meet other people, explore nature, and best of all, keeps you away from food!

There is a saying that goes something like, "If you want a different result, try a different approach." For those of you who have tried endless diets that haven't worked, why not try something that will? Asking yourself why you are eating, why you are choosing to put food into your mouth, at that moment and how you will feel if you do eat it: physically, emotionally, and spiritually, at the very least will slow down the eating process enough for you to mindfully decide whether eating the food in front of you is really the choice you want to make. Asking "Why am I eating this?" or a modified version of the question: "Why am I choosing to eat this right now?" can be the key that unlocks a whole new thin you. It can help you peel away the layers of mindless eating habits that are preventing you from being who you truly are.

I have spent most of my professional career training, counseling, guiding, listening, and watching as people address their health and lifestyle habits. I discovered that the people who were successful at losing weight were willing not only to change their eating and exercise patterns long-term but also to take a look at their unconscious habits, habits such as:

- Mindless eating
- Consuming excess portions
- Late-night snacking
- Indulging in high-fat snacks
- Eating nonstop without putting utensils down— or even pausing to breathe!

- Being a "closet eater" (believing that if no one is there to see you eat, it doesn't count)

I have learned that when people with these habits really paid attention to what they were eating—by keeping a food journal and noticing the patterns—suddenly, they found that they held the answers to their current weight issues. Their journal became their own personal diet book, and not something written by an "expert." They were able to see for themselves

 They had a lightbulb moment! They had found a whole new way to relate to food.

why the scale was not moving. Becoming aware of their habits, thoughts, and feelings around food actually turned on a light switch for them.

Food Traps

People frequently get into trouble when they don't recognize their food traps. A food trap is a situation that can cause you to eat more than you need to or more than you want to. It can be a time of day (4pm and you are tired) a social situation (a party where you don't know a lot of people and feel uncomfortable) special events (holiday celebration) or certain people (your significant other criticizes you around the house and you are angry.)

Clients who successfully lost weight became aware of their food traps and learned how to negotiate and plan for them. By identifying their food traps, they assumed control of what they ate so they could avoid self-sabotage and feel positive about themselves.

Case Study

Jim was a client who commuted one and a half hours each way to his sedentary desk job. He started becoming aware of his food traps of mindless snacking and portions that were way to large for his energy needs. His life turned around when he designed an "eating makcover" for himself. He cut out snacks on the way home from work when he was exhausted. He asked his wife to have more fruits and vegetables at home. He cut his portions in half. He also took up walking at least five days a week. But most importantly, he kept a food journal, taking note of everything he put in his mouth. He became aware of the food traps he had fallen into. Jim lost forty pounds and kept it off.

The goal of *Why Am I Eating This?* is to help you become aware of how your emotions and feelings affect your food intake. The exercises are designed to help you become aware of food traps and habits that subtly sabotage your efforts. These can be things such as types of food, times of day, emotional states, specific situations, certain people, types of events. Reading this book and answering the questions will launch you on a journey of self-awareness, fostering changes in your eating habits. The more aware you are when you are eating, the more your choices will start to be deliberate, thoughtful, and conscious. The more you contemplate your food traps and what you are feeling and when, the more you may start to notice spiritual and emotional hungers masquerading as physical hunger.

This book will facilitate the process, helping you inquire into the source of your frustrations and challenges with eating. It's a journey. The first step is to uncover what it is you are really craving. What's causing the sweet tooth? What kind of need is the candy bar filling in that moment; energy for your body or is it acting like an upper, which you feel will temporarily relieve an unpleasant emotion? Are you turning to food for:

- Comfort?
- Nurturing?
- Companionship?
- An escape?
- A creative outlet?
- Stuffing feelings?

Empowering Yourself with Choice

Remembering you always have choice when you are around food can be a helpful tip for you. This may seem obvious, but many students in my classes have realized that frequently they were eating for reasons outside of themselves. For example: someone else cooked and they wanted to please them, it is a social gathering and everyone else was eating, it was a cultural tradition in their circle, it was a certain time of day and everyone else was eating, they were at an "all you can eat buffet" and felt they should take full advantage of the spread. It was a "lightbulb" moment for many to realize they always a choice whether they put food in their mouth, no matter what others were doing around them. That is sometimes the hardest choice; saying "no" to food, even when everyone else is eating because you truly realize that your body does not need food in that moment.

As you read this book, you will have your own "lightbulb" moments as you begin to see your patterns of eating, understand where some of them came from, and decide to create your own new ways of eating healthfully that work for you.

It's all about choice: moment to moment.

You can choose to bypass the dangerous chocolate, potato chips, fries, pork rinds, ice cream, fudge, you-name-it beacon that's calling you, and choose instead to do somcthing else that truly nourishes you—or at least distracts you—whatever works to deter you and shift your attention to something else. Don't go into the kitchen, don't go by the secretary's desk with the bowl of chocolate; don't go near the vending machines at 4pm when you get the urge to eat. Choose an alternate path that does not include food in that moment!

Small habits make a difference. Small habits practiced day after day start to become permanent habits that can have huge results. When people start to see positive change, they feel successful, and this gives them confidence to keep going with this new habit. This is how "dieters" become long term healthy eaters. They realize they are not on a short, temporary course of change. They are changing their eating habits for a lifetime. They are changing their basic approach to food, every day.

 How do you want to change your basic approach to food: how you look at food, feel about food, what you think about food and what food you "go after"? What are all the small new choices you will now make?

Some examples of choosing a new approach to food: You can choose to take a very small bite and really taste it. You can chew deliberately and savor each bite. You can appreciate that you are eating chocolate, but you can take a smaller piece than you ordinarily would. You can change how you relate to, engage with, play games with, avoid, deny, or feel about your relationship with food.

How to Know It's Time for a Change

Sometimes we are angry, and we are so busy stuffing down feelings that we go unconscious and forget the amount we've eaten. And then we feel shame. How would it feel to avoid the shame and outwit your impulsive tendencies for immediate gratification instead?

Eating Mindfully: A Powerful Tool to Guide and Support You

"Mindfulness means paying attention in a particular way: on purpose, in the present moment, and nonjudgmentally." (Kabat-Zinn 1994) Mindful eating is a whole new way to approach food and life. Eating mindfully means eating with full attention and appreciation for what is in front of you, moment by moment. Often our minds and feelings are elsewhere when we eat, causing food to disappear.

Suddenly, we may think, "Where did that bag of chips go?" because while we were eating, we were daydreaming, worrying, reviewing the day, or planning for tomorrow. Or we are upset, depressed, or angry, and don't want to be, so we eat. Instead of the old way, mindful eating is eating with intention and chewing, tasting, and appreciating food in a new way.

Mindful eating is pausing, slowing down, putting our utensils on our plates in-between bites. Our full focus is on the food and being present with what we are eating, and with our company if we are eating with others. Sound boring? I have had clients tell me that just by shifting to mindful eating, pausing to breathe, eating with appreciation, and chewing their food many more times per bite, they have effortlessly lost ten to fifteen pounds. Others say they became aware of how often they were eating on impulse while listening to the TV or radio with no idea how much food they were consuming. They realized that eating mindfully helped them to change their whole approach to food: it helped them to slow down and to appreciate food in a new way. To look at food as fuel instead of just something to inhale. All of a sudden, they could see how often they were eating on automatic pilot.

Why Am I Eating This? will help you become victorious over food. You will masterfully gain control over your inner saboteurs. You will gain access to the power of choice and the courage to choose what serves you best. This book gives you an opportunity to change your life. You'll know you've reached the goal when you begin to think about what and why you're eating—before you open the cupboard door.

I Have Walked These Steps

I have struggled with my weight since childhood. I have had good years, when I kept my weight under control; great years, when I was exercising a lot, very happy in my work and personal life, and able to keep my weight ideal for me, and not-so-good years, when multiple stressors took over, causing me to eat more than I should in order to keep my energy up and feelings of fear and distress down. During those times, I was eating for many other reasons other than hunger: for comfort, company, distraction, or to ease my pain. At times food helped me celebrate. When there were deaths in my family, it gave me solace.

Even when people look at me and say, "You look great—you are thin," they are not aware of the internal struggles I still experience from time to time. Even an expert must remind him or herself of the traps that are easy to fall into if they return too often to food for reasons other than good nourishment and nutrition.

This is not to say that food cannot be used for celebratory purposes. But if we have grown up learning that "celebrate" means "to stuff yourself mercilessly" then it is time to learn a new strategy! When habits and emotions take over and we consume too much food for all the wrong reasons, that is when we can get into trouble.

I now use mindful eating as a tool for looking at eating and my relationship with food in an entirely new way. I use mindfulness to pause and eat much more slowly than those around me. I notice the textures and colors, aromas, and sensations from spices on my tongue in ways I never did before. I can witness the food and appreciate where it came from and the people who brought it to me. I can appreciate that it is on my plate, and I am fortunate to have it in front of me. I can mindfully and gratefully savor each bite, telling myself when I have had enough. I can say "STOP!" It is this approach that support me and allow me to look at food more neutrally, not as the demon it once was.

My personal experiences are woven in with what I have learned from hundreds of clients I have counseled and are condensed into seven basic steps for achieving weight-loss success. These are the steps that work for me and the steps that work for my clients. Each chapter in this book focuses on one of the steps.

Step 1: Self Awareness and Mindfulness
Step 2: Pay Attention
Step 3: Uncover the Mystery of Your Eating History
Step 4: Self Talk
Step 5: Gratitude
Step 6: Eating Light and Right for You
Step 7: Now what: Your New Eating Blueprint Starts Now!

There is no such thing as hearing the basics too many times. Some people may say "this is common sense" or "I already know this." You may know it but the statistics prove that people may have the knowledge but are not using it. Why? Perhaps their habits are not conscious. Perhaps they are unaware of how much they are eating. Perhaps they think the weight will magically go away if they want it to, especially if they know calorie counts. But it is really a question of math: burning more calories than you eat if you want to lose weight. My ninety-six-year-old father, who has been a disciplined eater his whole life, says, "It's as simple as remembering you must take in less food or exercise more." He has been a lifelong example to me of eating mindfully and stopping when he is full.

I have done informal research about what leads to diet success. People learn the basics of what they should eat: how to balance meals with food from all food groups, emphasizing protein, fruits, and vegetables (depending on what kind of diet their bodies feel comfortable with) and of course, adding exercise. They learn to read labels, learn to cut portions in half; learn about hidden fats, sugar, and salt. They learn about the empty calories in junk food. They learn about portion control and how the average dinner portion in a restaurant is two or three servings, sometimes more. But after that, it always comes down to one really big secret: how successful people are with their food intake is really a function of their minds and discipline. It is a function of their will to say no to food, even though they may feel that they really want it at the time. It means they are equipped with the tools to look at food as a nutrient, not as a drug to numb; they are able to pause and choose what foods, how much food, and even if they truly want to eat, deliberately.

No matter how hard you have struggled or how many times you have failed, it is possible to train your mind to look at food differently and be empowered around food. What a concept: you have control over food, instead of it controlling you!

 I can control how I approach food instead of it controlling me.

I Have Heard Stories

In my career managing corporate wellness programs and in my consulting mind-body practice, I have worked with hundreds of individuals, and the ones who followed all seven steps lost weight and kept it off. The ones who did the best took time to focus on their food behavior and emotions in addition to calories and portions. They noticed the times of the day they would fall into eating traps, such as after work and late in the evening, when boredom, anxiety, or loneliness set in. Many kept track of these challenging moments and planned in advance by having fresh fruit, veggies, hot-air popcorn, or other low-fat, high-fiber snacks ready. They learned to take a walk or to call a friend when the urge to eat struck. Some found that paying bills was a good distraction: all their hands were occupied! Keeping a food journal seemed to help them be more aware of calories consumed, especially when they were honest enough to write down even one cracker, piece of hard candy or stick of gum.

Sometimes it can be difficult to make it through all seven steps. Some of my clients have made it successfully through steps one to four and hit a wall at step five. They found it hard to be grateful for small amounts of food; that felt like deprivation to them. They couldn't get over the hump of visually being satisfied with less on their plate. Psychologically they felt something had been taken away and they did not want to practice using their minds in a more conscious way. Others didn't believe they could create new permanent eating patterns that would last into the future and/or they didn't know how. They were afraid to visualize a scene in the future where they could be satisfied with less food. They didn't believe they could say no to food, based on their failures to say no in the past. But once they started to practice envisioning the positive changes they would make, and what it would look and feel like to choose food deliberately, they were on a new path to a new way of eating.

Sometimes it is not easy to get started. Readiness is important. People who are not ready cannot change any behavior, whether it is stopping smoking or changing eating habits. You have to be ready! Are you ready?

Being ready means being willing to do whatever it takes. It means you have a high level of intention to accomplish your goal, no matter what the obstacle or sacrifice.

Other clients did not know how to invent strategies for nourishing themselves. They had no idea what that meant, or they didn't know where to start. When I later asked them to think of actions that represented self-care and being good to themselves—something unrelated to food that made them feel good, positive, and comforted—they understood. They realized that connecting with friends or family, rest, water, lighting a candle, making a fire, time spent focusing on nature, time spent with a pet, pausing for five minutes of silence, focusing on breathing, or praying, meditating, or taking a meditative walk, could be calming, supportive, and could take the edge off their belief that food was always the answer. But it does take practice.

Others have realized that when they ate, they were thinking of other things or zoning out—they really had no idea how much they were eating because they were not paying attention to amount of food. Their minds were far away.

Some clients felt that if they activated their new blueprint and went back to their old eating ways for a few days that they were doomed to failure. It was all or nothing. They were afraid to make the commitment to begin, for fear of failure. But once they remembered that life is a series of twists and turns and that we can always begin anew, they were willing to say, "OK, I'm willing to begin this new journey, exploring my relationship with food, moment to moment."

Each of us is unique; everyone assimilates things differently. *Why Am I Eating This?* is the result of extensive health counseling, background, research, and personal life experiences. Take each step of the seven-step process and use the wisdom in each chapter in your own way and start to put your struggles with weight behind you.

A Meditation:

Take a breath. Take another breath. From a quiet space, try to imagine that you have everything you need: all is perfect in your life. There is no need to push, to cajole, to struggle, to manipulate, to want. From this perfect place, imagine there is a sumptuous buffet in front of you. Everything you can imagine is there: all types, varieties, shapes, and sizes of the best food on earth, emitting delectable aromas. You are given a plate. People will serve you. How much will you choose? How much food do you really want when you have everything you need on all levels? You have enough to nourish your body right now. You don't need to worry about the next meal because you know you will be provided for; see yourself taking just enough, but not too much. Feel the feeling of satisfaction knowing that you have all the nourishment you need.

CHAPTER TWO

DISCOVER YOUR FOOD PATTERNS:
PAY ATTENTION

- What if it were possible to unlock the secret of why we eat what we do?
- What if it were possible to change conditioned behaviors and thought patterns associated with food?
- What if it were possible to lose weight, not with deprivation, but by looking at food in a different way and loving your true self?
- What if it were possible to leave the past behind and create a new you?

The first step in redesigning your eating blueprint begins with discovering your current blueprint and why you're still trapped by your automatic- eating habits. Discovery requires paying attention to your relationship with food from a mindful perspective.

The American Heritage College Dictionary defines attention as "concentration of the mental powers, a close observing or listening." When this definition is applied to the process of eating, the phrase "to pay attention" means to be mindful of what is underneath your desire to eat; be aware of what you are eating, acknowledge how delicious each bite tastes, and be grateful for each bite.

Mindfulness, introduced in the first chapter, is a way of paying attention in the moment, a way of attending to what, in our mind, hearts, and souls, is affecting what we are choosing to eat and when. People spend thousands of dollars on therapy to deal with their weight problems and still never figure out the answers. Ruth Quillian-Wolever, PhD, was interviewed by Kelly McCabe and said, "Mindfulness differs from behavior therapy in that mindfulness is attending to the inner world—thought, emotional behavior." (Quillian-Wolever 2007) Paying attention to our inner world, moment to moment, is really the answer we have been seeking.

Behavioral psychology teaches that bringing unconscious thoughts or feelings to the conscious mind is the first step toward changing our behavior. Knowing why we do what we do gives us a new awareness and power over our choices. Being conscious of why and when we put food in our mouths will help us to uncover the secrets to solving our eating problems and our struggles with weight.

Jean Kristeller, PhD, a renowned researcher with expertise in addiction and behavioral change, has received two NIH grants to teach and evaluate a Mindfulness-Based Eating Awareness Training (MB-EAT) at Indiana State. It has also been piloted at other universities including Duke and the University of Pennsylvania. In an interview with Richard Mahler, she says, "Habits are conditioning, and conditioning affects every aspect of our lives ... habits affect our choices of food, our preferences, the amount we eat, when we eat and how we eat ... with mindfulness, they can step back, observe, and introduce a moment of choice. With mindfulness, they can choose to eat consciously." (Kristeller 2005) Eating mindfully gives us more awareness and appreciation for the taste of each bite we take.

We savor our food so much more when we eat mindfully.

When we are mindful, we are putting all our attention on the present moment, without rushing and without our thoughts being elsewhere. We are in the present. We take in the beauty around us, the pleasantness of the company we are with, but our thoughts and awareness stay in present time. Taking in the surroundings and company helps to expand the feeling of being nourished by the environment and others. Then the process of eating becomes a multisensory experience; you are not looking to your food to nourish you on all levels; you are taking in the sensory experience and allowing that to nourish you. Notice how often your thoughts are all over the place when you are eating. Mindfulness helps to slow you down and direct your attention to stay with one thought and one activity, the process of eating and savoring each bite.

The Secret Meaning of Food

For most of us, the "meaning of food" is a foreign concept. When I've asked students in a class about what food means to them, they generally say "I like it." We're used to having food in front of us and eating it—whatever's there, whenever we want it. When it comes to food, most of us are on autopilot. We don't think about what we are eating or why; we just grab and go! Often, we are in a hurry or caught up in the moment of conversation or celebration. We have never been trained to contemplate food with each bite or why we eat as much as we do ... meals were to be eaten, not to be thought about.

When we were growing up, perhaps certain foods were withheld when we were young, or perhaps there was never enough of it. So, when it's available now, it controls us. For example, we get a box of candy as a gift and soon the box is empty. After all, it's a gift; it must be eaten. Or maybe my family will eat it all and there won't be any left if I don't eat it all now. Maybe as children we were told what we could and couldn't eat. So now we eat whatever we want as fast as we can. For some people, food can mean other things: a symbol of being loved, a symbol of being nurtured, and a symbol of being cared for. Maybe the only time we were happy was when we were around food, which numbed us to the unhappy circumstances and moods around us.

 What does food mean to me?

As an adult, my passion for studying and teaching about the mind-body connection has allowed me to experience the power of my mind in all things, including food intake. I have learned that dieting is, in many ways, a mind game.

As a child, I had terrible struggles with food. My mother would cook my favorite meal whenever there was something to celebrate. There would be tons of food, followed by a rich dessert. I wanted to please her and show my appreciation, so I always ate a lot more than I really needed. Food equaled love. Frequently my mother was the happiest and nicest to me when she was cooking and serving food. I associated food with happiness.

On the other side of the spectrum, food could go beyond love, nurturing, and caring to a level of anesthesia. In my family, when there was upset in our lives, we ate to make ourselves feel better. If people were angry, they ate a lot. And grazed in the kitchen constantly. Rich, plentiful food numbed us to any unpleasantness.

If a friend or family member was gravely ill, we ate. Eating took the place of feeling.

It took years, but I finally figured out that I wasn't the only one who used food in at least two useless ways. The first was as a distraction that allowed me to avoid doing or feeling something that I perceived as unpleasant. The second useless way I was using food was as an emotional buffer, to avoid feeling my real feelings. If I felt angry, sad, frustrated, impatient, or that things were out of control, it was much easier to stuff my face with popcorn or chips than to feel the feelings. The combination of several mindfulness and mind-body trainings helped me to be aware of what I was feeling—or avoiding feeling. Eating a raisin mindfully at Harvard's Institute for Mind Body Medicine woke up my sense that there was another way to approach food...slowly and thoughtfully. Through the years, courses in various forms of meditation also allowed me to practice feeling uncomfortable and to avoid using food to stop the discomfort.

This was a new way of living for me. Practicing being still and present in the silence, and just "being," with nothing to do but to stay aware in the midst of the discomfort, frustration, or anger, allowed me to see that I could handle the emotion instead of it handling me. It also showed me that overeating was just a result of not wanting to feel discomfort. It also was because my thoughts were stuck in frustration and a sense of helplessness. In that detour, food was a friend that kept me company while I hung out in a sense of helplessness. I learned that I could handle it if I was just willing to think a positive thought that would lead to a positive action, such as "I can do this." The second step was to practice patience, mindfulness, and gratitude. By taking these actions steps, I learned I could stay aware of my feelings instead of stuffing them. Best of all, I felt empowered rather than helpless.

Where are our thoughts and feelings when we are eating? Are we eating with appreciation and gratitude, or zoning out, thinking about the past or the future? How many times have you stood in the kitchen with a spoon, eating right out of a container of ice cream, instead of doing paperwork? How many times have you gorged on chocolate instead of phoning your friend to apologize for harsh words you didn't really mean? How many times have you felt you had to eat something really bad while you did your taxes because you saw it as a reward for doing something that was painful? Snacking numbed the frustration and made the task less tedious. Gorging was a reward for standing up to the challenge. Whatever the reason, becoming aware of why and when we are eating helps us to change the habit. The problem is, we gorge away our pain, anger, and upset, but after the numbness goes away, we are left with other feelings that are actually worse: guilt, shame, and regret. But at the time, it seemed worth it.

How I use food for the wrong reasons.

 "In other words, do I really want/ need to eat this right now?"

Lately, I have noticed that my hunger is frequently related to frustration. If a task seems particularly challenging or complicated, I feel an overwhelming sense of "I can't do this" come over me. Then I want to eat. I have noticed that if I just pause, remember that I can do it, breathe, and continue, breathe, and continue, the waves of hunger go away.

It's time to tune in to your body and feel what's really going on when you believe you are "hungry." And it could be that you are thirsty. We don't drink enough water during the day, and when we feel our energy is low, we assume we are hungry. Try drinking a few glasses of water and reassessing your hunger. If you still think you are hungry, be willing to pause, look within, and feel anger, sadness, happiness, or loneliness. Feel the entire range of your emotions, rather than anesthetizing them with food. Be aware of when you turn to food for any reason other than genuine hunger. Sometimes drinking a cup of water or tea, and/or having a piece of fruit helps. But I have also noticed that I need to avoid the trap of escaping uncomfortable feelings by stuffing them, procrastinating, or pretending they are not there. Actually, telling myself that I can do it, and taking it one small step at a time helps.

Some people do not want to feel an empty stomach. To them, this might feel scary. They may have a fear there is not enough food available and they may starve. This might be because of a childhood memory or something else. But to them an empty stomach is a bad thing. (Diabetics might start to sense their blood sugar is dropping when their stomachs feel empty, but this is different, and most diabetics have been trained to eat every few hours and to carry healthy snacks with them, so they are always prepared.)

Clients who took themselves through the seven steps successfully said the more aware, or conscious, they stayed while they were eating—even adding such little steps as saying, "Thank you for this food," and "I am mindfully eating," or "I am choosing to eat this now"—helped them to pace themselves and enjoy their food even more. They also noticed that the more grateful they stayed, savoring each bite, the less they ate. The focus was on appreciating the food instead of going on automatic pilot or stuffing their feelings.

How do you do this?

For those of you who have never pondered your inner feelings, have no desire to do so, or think it doesn't matter, there is still hope. Most of us do have a sense of how much food is enough from a practical viewpoint. We can tell from when we have been under stress and lost or gained weight, how much we ate. Or when we went on a "diet" and were able to really limit our calories, how much was "enough." But then people get lazy and forget that feeling of "this is enough-its time to stop eating."

So, when you are eating more than you know you need, just stop and ask "why?" Make up your own questions to ask yourself, such as:

- How much is enough?
- Do I need this?
- Is it helpful?
  Will I feel crummy after eating it?
- What purpose will it serve?
- How many calories am I ingesting?
- Am I even hungry right now?

A way to remind yourself to assess what is really going on before you eat is to test your hunger level. Simply say to yourself "How hungry am I"? This scale, from 1 to 4, works by reminding you how physically hungry you are. This guides you to be honest with yourself about how much food you really need right now, separate from the psychological or emotional cravings you might be having. You might say that you are:

1. Not hungry
2. Mildly hungry
3. Hungry
4. Famished

If you find that your hunger is not physical, pause for a moment and ask yourself:

- What is really going on right now?
- Why do I want to eat?
- Am I bored?
- Do I just want a distraction from what I am doing?
- What else might I be craving—connection, friendship, attention, reassurance?

Dieticians recommend keeping a food journal where you combine 3 steps: what you ate (down to how many crackers, pretzels, or cookies) how hungry you were and your emotional state. Keeping a food journal, quite simply, keeps you honest. It allows you to monitor your eating patterns, and to see trends related to situations, times of day and emotional states.

Some other questions you may want to ponder. These questions will help you get to know yourself and look at why you are choosing food other than because you are hungry, and you need fuel. See if a pattern is developing. Focus. Pay attention. Be aware. It will pay off in the end.

- Am I uncomfortable in a new or stressful situation? Do I feel frustrated, angry, sad, or lonely?

- Am I fulfilled in my relationships with other people? Do I feel disappointed in myself or others?
- Why am I eating something that will make me drowsy? Why am I eating when I am not hungry?
- Am I eating this now because I am depressed?
- Why am I eating this so quickly?
- Am I angry with myself?
- Am I mad at someone?
- Do I feel out of control?
- Am I eating this because I am tired?
- Am I eating this because I'm nervous or scared? Do I feel confused?
- Do I feel jealous? Do I feel guilty?
- Am I eating this now because I am frustrated with things not changing in my life, no matter how hard I try?
- Am I eating this now because I think it will give me energy?
- What is it that I am really seeking?

This is an opportunity for what psychologists have termed "self-talk," the words we say to ourselves all day long. Self-talk can be very valuable in helping us stick to our program. It can guide us and keep us on track. It is part of the process of "paying attention" as we notice our thoughts when we are around food. Instead of a friend being there to ask us questions about what is going on, or to re-direct our thoughts or attention to other things, self-talk can act as our own internal coach. It's not just a question of programming ourselves with positive affirmations. They can be helpful but may sound rote after a while if you are walking into the kitchen saying "I am a thin person" as you are heading to the ice-cream. Instead, self-talk can guide us in the moment; ask questions, give answers. It can give us a lot of insight and help us to pause to control our impulses and re-choose a healthier option.

Dr. Martin Seligman, Ph.D., director of the Positive Psychology Center at the University of Pennsylvania, has written about and studied explanatory style and optimism for years. Explanatory style is how we explain things that are happening to us and in our lives, moment by moment. It is our own internal coach that may serve to guide us in the right direction or sabotage us if our patterns of thought tend to be self-defeating. Self-talk is important because it is the words, we say to ourselves when we are upset. (More on self-talk in Chapter 4) As he says, explanatory style is especially important because it reflects how we explain setbacks or challenges. Do we go into a victim mentality, telling ourselves, "This always happens to me," or do we remind ourselves that this happens to other people too and we are not alone in facing a challenge? Do we tell ourselves it is a permanent situation or a temporary one? Can we isolate our frustration to this one area of our life, or do we label ourselves as failures in all aspects of our life because we are having a little setback in this one area? This connects with food intake and dieting in several important ways: when we want to eat but know we shouldn't, self-talk and explanatory style can be the strength that guides us out of a challenging place, back into a neutral zone of "What do I want to focus on right now?" It can be humorous and funny; it doesn't have to be serious. The point is that your own deliberate self-talk can help you to re-frame the situation quickly, so that you are alert enough to guide your thoughts and therefore your actions to a conscious, healthy choice.

For example, if you tend to generalize when you are on a diet, saying things to yourself like:

"I never can win at dieting; I'm a failure at this like in everything in life," it would be helpful to insert a more helpful thought such as:

"I can do this, one step at a time. This is one thing I can take charge of in my life."

Going Underneath the Surface

When you face the feelings that lie underneath the urge to eat, it is an opportunity to face your cravings in an entirely new way. In that moment, is food acting as a source to fill authentic hunger, a drug to satiate emotional hunger, or an avoidance mechanism? You know the answer. Every time you eat, you have the opportunity to create a new vision of yourself—just for you, not to please or impress anyone else.

You can show yourself that you have control over your actions and your life—*You have the power to take control!*

Exercise 1: Part A

Over the next few days, rate your hunger before you eat, on a scale from 1 to 4, "1" being not very hungry, to "4" being very hungry. Notice how many times a day you are eating when your actual hunger level is low. In the second exercise, you will go into more detail by asking yourself why: is it a stall tactic, boredom, or something else? Notice your emotions and

feelings. And if you are willing, write down your thoughts when you feel the urge to eat.

Exercise 1: Part B

The following exercise will help you understand why you are eating and when. The goal of the exercise is to help you get in the habit of thinking about what and why you are eating, as well as the real triggers for your trip to the refrigerator or fast-food restaurant, other than true physical hunger.

Ask yourself these questions before you eat:

1. Why am I eating this; am I truly hungry? (If not, perhaps I'm sad, lonely, frustrated, anxious, depressed, angry, etc.)
2. If I am not hungry, what is it that really want right now? What is it that I really am craving? (Company, an easier life, a place where I belong, more friends, happiness)
3. Is this food going to get me there? (You know the answer.)

Some people call it discipline; some people call it deprivation. I call it honoring and caring for yourself. Look at this conscious process as an entirely new way of living. Learning to say no to food when you are not hungry is easier when you envision the body and health that reflects who you really are. Learn to say "yes" to loving and respecting yourself.

I have had clients use this technique, with their own variations of these questions, and it really works. Some have added the mindfulness technique of breathing and pausing, quieting themselves, and going within. They report that breathing techniques help them to center themselves and get focused on their real goal at the moment. Frequently they are able to choose a healthy alternative to a fattening snack or just walk away from the kitchen.

I know that when I practice this, I find myself talking into the refrigerator, asking, "What am I really looking for right now—what is it that I really want?" Soon, I realize that what I am seeking at the moment is not in the refrigerator! Other people have had similar reactions:

> Ted, on one of his late-evening grazes, goes to the refrigerator, opens the door, and stares inside. Instead of helping himself to a piece of cake left over from dessert, he chooses fresh fruit.

> Liz, feeling nervous at a party, goes for more of the veggies and salad instead of high-fat cheese and crackers, which used to be her standby favorites.

> At the celebration party at work, Tom, who is working on changing his habits, takes a small piece of brownie, and eats it very slowly, feeling satisfied with a small amount.

A Meditation:

Imagine yourself at a party where there is a medley of food laid out, all your favorites. There are main courses, salads, vegetables, side dishes, fresh fruit, and sumptuous desserts. Picture yourself scanning the whole table first to get a sense of what is there. Then watch yourself check in with yourself to see how hungry, on a scale of 1–4, you really are at this time. You are aware that your hunger is at a "2." Then see yourself mentally choosing ahead of time what you will take and what portion size you will choose. You see that the portions are small, yet you have a sampling of several of your favorite items. Then imagine yourself tasting each thing slowly, chewing deliberately, and taking the time to appreciate the food and where it came from. Simultaneously, you take in the surroundings and the people you are with, and perhaps you engage in conversation. You notice that you are pacing yourself, not rushing, but taking more time than you normally would so that you can savor your food and really taste each bite. See yourself taking at least twenty minutes to finish what is on your plate. Then imagine that you realize you are fully satisfied and do not need any more food at this time. You know that if you want to have more food later, it will be there for you. You are happy to turn your attention to the guests, sip a beverage slowly, and enjoy the party.

CHAPTER THREE

UNCOVER THE MYSTERY OF
YOUR EATING HISTORY

- Why do I love to eat?
- Why do I eat when I'm sad?
- Why do I eat when food is put in front of me, whether or not I'm hungry?
- Why does the word "celebration" trigger "all-you-can-eat" in my mind?
- Why do I try to force second and third portions on my guests, just like my mother did?

In an attempt to answer these and other questions, we need to explore our personal eating history. We each come with our own unique history and conditioning regarding food, which very often dictates who we are today, how we eat, and how we live our lives. This is what we call our "eating blueprint." For example, if I were to answer the above questions, my answers might look something like:

1. I love to eat because I feel happy when I eat, no matter what is going on. It may be either a communal or a solitary experience, each with different benefits. It is instant gratification, no matter where I am.

2. I eat when I'm sad because when I do so, temporarily, I don't feel sad anymore. My attention is on the food and the feel of comfort I get as I am eating. It fills me up. But I realize this is just a temporary gain. The sadness inevitably comes back if I don't take a look at why I feel sad.

3. I have been conditioned from my childhood to eat whenever food was there. It was what you did; no one ever really thought about it. My father was the only one in the family who was very disciplined; he exercised a lot and could afford extra calories. Instead, he often said no to food, even when everyone else at the table was indulging. Watching him was the first place I learned you could say "no" to food, even on holiday occasions when everyone else was eating "just because" it seemed like that was the ritual.

4. Celebrations meant "eat, eat, eat" in my family. There was always plenty of special food—and huge portions. The underlying message was that it was OK, and we were even expected to eat a lot at a celebratory event.

5. I try to force second and third portions on my guests because that is what my mother did—but I hated when she did that! I do it because, underneath, I know she was trying to be generous and hospitable, and in some ways, I still want to be like her. Perhaps this goes back to the "food equals love" message. However, I also know that sometimes it felt like coercion.

We are constantly flooded with new rules for eating the "right" way in order to be seen as attractive in American culture. We are inundated with messages in books, magazines, movies, and on TV. We are bombarded with images of size-two models and lean, mean men with little body fat and "six pack abs"—and a multitude of suggestions for how to look like them.

The idea of everyone being a size two or having "six-pack abs" belies the fact that who we are is a combination of our ethnic and social conditioning, our genetic disposition, and our cultural background. In fact, looking like a model goes against many people's metabolic makeup. In subscribing to these ideals, we are striving to duplicate a prototype which may go against the very nature of who we are and where we've come from. We may better understand ourselves by discovering our own personal food history, taking into account any cultural messages specific to our generation or ethnic background, we can better understand our own personal perspective in this area.

If it is your genetic or cultural background to be big boned, it is likely that you were not meant to be rail thin. If your ancestors were braving the wild elements in Nordic climates, it could be that you were meant to have some meat on you. Psychologist William Sheldon has classified people into three main body types: the ectomorph, the mesomorph, and the endomorph. According to WorldFitness.org, "The ectomorph has a short upper body, long arms and legs, long narrow feet and hands and very little fat storage. Narrow shoulders and narrow chest with long thin muscles ... The mesomorph has a large chest, long torso, solid muscle mass and is very strong. Mesomorphs find it easy to build muscle mass and respond well to training of all types ... The endomorph has short musculature, a round face, short neck, wide hips, and heavy fat storage. Endomorphs will not have trouble building muscle mass but will have trouble losing fat." Do you know what body type you are?

Remembering my culinary heritage, how it was passed on from my grandmother to my mother and how it influenced so much of my childhood was the beginning of liberating myself from my past. This doesn't mean I don't still cherish German pfefferneusse, springerles, and stollen at Christmastime, or nice Scottish shortbread at a party, but I choose carefully and deliberately, instead of loading up my plate. Sometimes a taste of something is just as satisfying as a whole serving. Or, maybe just looking at these items is enough. I can recall all the fond memories of parents, grandparents, and aunts gathered together partaking in these delights. But I don't have to necessarily eat the sweets to recall the memory, with happiness. And if I do have some, I have learned to ask myself the question, "How much is enough?" while I am eating.

 Even at a celebration, asking "How much is enough?" means I can still enjoy the party, but I don't have to equate more food with more fun.

I've learned the amount of food I consume at a celebration doesn't affect my happiness quotient. They are not interdependent! This realization, of course, came after years of stuffing myself and not feeling particularly good the next day. I have realized over time that as I was growing up, "celebration" was equated with pigging out. I recalled fun, happy times, and it seemed that the more people ate, the happier they were. Of course, I realize now that it was all temporary. The temporary highs from sugar and carbohydrate binging came back to haunt me the next day. "Celebration" conjures up different things in each person's mind. What does it mean to you? Each of you has a story that created your eating blueprint, and it's of vital importance to discover what that story is.

Several of my clients and I have experienced overeating that was generated by spite. For me, the trigger was my mother. She would prepare heavy, fancy meals, and then wonder why I wasn't thin. She would say things such as, "Maybe you should spend some more time caring about your looks and batting your eyelashes." This made me so furious that I promptly stuffed my face. I remember countless times when my mother said something that would set me off, but I didn't have any healthy outlet for my anger and rage—I didn't know what to do with it. So, I would stuff it, partly to get back at my mother. "Oh, you want me to be thin, do you?" And I would eat more. Several female clients have told me they eat out of spite: toward a mother, father, husband, or friend. Because they believe that someone wants them to do something, namely, to be thin, they are so angry that they do the opposite. While this may make sense on some levels, this argument fails because the ultimate outcome is a feeling of failure and shame. Take a walk. Breathe. Do not let them get you down. Care for yourself, give yourself some love, and nourish yourself in other ways that will help you heal from the harmful words of others.

The following exercise will help you discover your eating history, similar to those I have just described. The goal is for you to discover how many unconscious eating patterns are related to your childhood: what you saw, heard, and experienced growing up.

Exercise 2

In this exercise, write down any memories from your childhood connecting food, feelings and weight issues. It could be something someone said to you or something you observed at family gatherings. Were you offered a sweet snack when you arrived? Were you served and encouraged to eat large portions, because that was being generous? What was the atmosphere like at your childhood dinner table: peaceful, angry, confrontational, or frantic? Did you have a chance to speak? Was your voice heard? Did you come to the table upset from conversations that took place when you got home? Were you encouraged to eat as much as you cared to or forced to clean your plate? Were you rewarded with special dinners or desserts?

Write down anything you can think of. As you write, be aware of any insights or emotions that may surface. Write those down as they come up. This is an opportunity to really get in touch with where you come from, and it might provide some very valuable clues to your eating history. You may suddenly understand where some of your habits and tendencies toward food originated.

My memories of food and my family:

By taking a few quiet moments to understand some of your history around food, you've started laying a foundation for discovering your current eating blueprint. Now the trick is to stay mindful of your eating history, particularly at large gatherings where it may be so influential.

Set goals for yourself for example:

1. When I'm at parties, I will stay away from the food table.
2. I will think twice about tasting all the food on the buffet table just because it's in front of me.
3. I will ask myself three times if I really need a second helping.
4. If I have to have dessert, I will share one, even though my heritage was known for its exceptional sweet treats, and frequently I find myself thinking that's how I grew up, so I'm entitled to eat sweets.
5. Just because everyone else is gorging themselves doesn't mean I have to do the same. I can engage in conversation; help clear the table or wash the dishes; anything to distract myself from wanting to eat more.

A Meditation:

Take a few full, deep breaths and settle into a quiet, calm space that is free of intruding thoughts and interruptions. Picture yourself at the next family gathering where there is a medley of all of your favorite foods from childhood. See them laid out beautifully, wonderful aromas coming from the special foods. Imagine that you look over them and quietly decide ahead of time which ones you must taste and which ones you can leave behind; leave to your memories. Picture yourself going down the line of the buffet table and taking small portions of the things that are most important to you.

You know you can always go back for more if you really want it. Now see yourself taking slow, mindful bites of each dish, appreciating with gratitude the special tastes that evoke warm, happy memories. As you chew each bite slowly, really tasting the food, you are happy to be tasting it from a new perspective, with appreciation, instead of inhaling it like you normally would. Picture yourself taking at least twenty minutes to eat what is on your plate, knowing it takes at least that long for it to register in your brain when you are full.

After twenty minutes, you contemplate if you really want more. After one small taste of your most favorite dish of your most favorite dish, you realize you are full, you are complete. You feel good and proud you did not overeat, that you enjoyed and ate at this celebration with care and deliberation, with a great outcome. And you now know you can do it again. You will take these tools with you to the next celebration or dining out experience.

CHAPTER FOUR

SELF-TALK:
BRIDGING THE GAP

- When I am around food, what am I saying to myself?
- Why, as soon as food is put in front of me, do I immediately want more, before I have even tasted anything?
- When I eat with others, what am I saying to myself?
- If others go for second helpings, what is my response?
- If people around me are eating fast, what do I say to myself?

Most people, especially if they have dieted in the past, know what to eat and what not to eat to lose weight. The problem is not the lack of knowledge.

The problem is bridging the gap between their intellectual knowledge of "good food and bad food" and controlling their behavior when they are around food, especially when they are not hungry.

I'm offering a way to bridge the gap between these two powerful forces: knowledge and behavior.

The bridge consists of 1) noticing your thought patterns and emotions whenever you are around food, and staying aware of how negative ones can sabotage your efforts. 2) As a result of monitoring your thoughts and feelings, have your next steps be deliberate actions aligned with your goals of a healthy you. When you are able to notice your automatic thoughts around food, insert healthy, positive ones, and link your actions to those healthy, positive thoughts, you will be on the road to success. This will make the difference in your life between a temporary diet where you gain the weight back and a permanent, sustainable change in the way you approach food that will last for a lifetime.

Part of this bridge is zeroing in on your thoughts in more detail, especially the messages you are constantly saying to yourself throughout the day, both positive and negative. And noticing the emotions or situations that seem to trigger you. If you notice a pattern like "I seem to give in to food when I feel frustrated," start practicing an alternate healthy behavior such as breathing, taking a walk, calling a friend, or saying something positive like "no problem."

As mentioned earlier in Chapter 2, this messaging to self is known as "self-talk" in the psychological world.

"We all talk to ourselves all the time; it is how we frame our worlds." (Seligman 1990) This is how the "father of positive psychology" explains the basis of noticing our self-talk, moment to moment, and how that can change our lives. In *Learned Optimism*, he wrote eloquently, describing how people have turned their lives around by changing the way they frame each situation in their lives. Dr. Seligman asks people to contemplate if they are an optimist or a pessimist, and to look at how they explain setbacks to themselves. Both of these key questions and the answers are important because they can alter a downward spiral of negativity. He calls it your "explanatory style," which in essence, is how you interpret and frame your life.

We see in his powerful book that our moment-to-moment thoughts have moment-to-moment consequences.

Our self-talk has a direct connection with our actions. Often, people do not learn healthy ways to redirect their minds' chatter. Instead, they learn unhealthy coping behaviors to handle their hurts, pains, and frustrations. We have a tendency to say, "I am the way that I am, I can't change." However, research has shown that you can literally change your mind and your thought patterns by substituting new, deliberate, helpful and supportive thoughts to change the quality of your life in each moment.

Dr. Seligman's approach is based on cognitive behavioral therapy (CBT), a form of psychotherapy developed by Aaron Beck, MD at the University of Pennsylvania. CBT hit the mainstream in 1970 with a book by David Burns, MD, *Feeling Good: The New Mood Therapy*.

Dr. Burns simplified the concept so that anyone could understand the concept of cognitive distortions, and the way in which our thoughts sometimes distort reality for us. By recognizing the distortions as they happen and inserting other, more helpful, affirming thoughts, we can change our moods and change our actions to healthy ones.

Dr. Burns asks us to challenge our thoughts in every moment. By asking ourselves if we are "overgeneralizing," "jumping to conclusions," or "disqualifying the positive," we can identify how we sabotage ourselves in our daily lives, leading to a downward spiral of thoughts, feelings, emotions, and actions. When we relate this to eating, we start seeing that our thoughts and emotions influence our actions when we are around food. If we can challenge negative thoughts and remind ourselves to keep affirming positive, deliberate thoughts, it can help us to navigate through challenging times when all we want to do is resort to our old, destructive eating behaviors.

According to a 2005 press release by the University of Pennsylvania, research by Dr. Aaron Beck, MD showed cognitive therapy to work at least as well as antidepressant drug therapy in all respects, and cognitive therapy showed more lasting effects. This does not mean that you should throw out your antidepressants; consult your medical doctor about this issue. Rather, it shows the power of learning how to challenge and change your negative thoughts when they pop up during the day. Over time, negative thoughts and moods can not only affect your mood but your self-esteem. "Feeling Good: The New Mood Therapy" (Burns: 1970) gave many examples and case histories of people who were able to connect the way they think to the way they feel and turn their lives around. The bottom line: people with high self-esteem practice healthy behaviors. They feel good about who they are so they practice self-care.

Both experts in challenging our thoughts and inserting new, helpful ones, Dr. Seligman and Dr. Burns, have contributed much to the field of psychology. They teach people that we can retrain our minds in new, positive, helpful ways that can influence our behaviors, including habits related to health, including food intake. We can use their work by staying conscious and mindful and using positive self-talk when we are around food. Disciplined eaters who manage their weight also manage their self-talk when they're around food. For example, they may say some variation of the following to themselves:

"Just because it's there doesn't mean I have to eat it." "I'm not hungry."

"It is made of fat."

"It is made of sugar."

It is pure carbohydrate, which will make me drowsy." "I just ate an hour ago."

"I've had enough. I can walk away from the food now." "Eat slowly, pause, and appreciate each bite."

"Take time to stop and breathe. Put my utensils down and pause." "Just because everyone around me is pigging out doesn't mean I have to."

"It is time to stop."

"As I pause to think about it, I'm not really hungry right now."

Harvard's Institute for Mind Body Medicine focuses on the power of the mind-body connection in their eight-week classes on everything from heart disease to cancer to back pain to healthy living. One of the foundations of all their programs is cognitive restructuring; making people aware of their thought patterns and teaching them how to insert helpful, instead of sabotaging, messages to themselves. In terms of food, we are frequently unaware of all the messages we are sending ourselves. Whether it is positive, "I will have something healthy now," or negative, "I'm frustrated, so what does it matter how much I eat."? what we say to ourselves right before eating often dictates what we put into our mouths.

So, if some of our self-talk is helpful and some of our self-talk is not, why not choose the option that's positive or constructive? This will guide us in a healthy direction. Plus, it's something we always have with us: our ability to choose our thoughts.

Diagram of Self-talk Outcomes:

> **Frustration → Negative self-talk →**
> **More frustration → Negative behavior**
>
> **versus**
>
> **Frustration → Positive self-talk → Enhanced**
> **self-esteem and peace → Healthy behavior**

Remember that mindfulness is slowing down to appreciate each moment with gratitude and appreciation. Some examples of mindful self-talk that can lead to healthy eating behaviors:

"I am mindfully aware that this is enough."

"I have plenty to eat; one bite at a time."

"This small amount nourishes me and fills me up."

"I can always have more later."

"I have plenty and I am satisfied as I take in this food and my surroundings with appreciation."

As we discussed in chapter one, sometimes we find ourselves saying, "I'm hungry," when really what we are feeling is:

"I'm tired."

"I'm angry."

"I'm frustrated."

This calls for our best self-talk to kick in and give us the antidote for the downward spiral that is about to kick in.

Saying, "Stop, BREATHE, pause, and re-choose," as we take a deep breath will give us the time to rethink our decisions.

 Managing our self-talk by monitoring and interrupting negative thoughts and inserting positive ones is a way to navigate our way to a healthy choice. It is a way to feel empowered.

Another aspect of self-talk is gratitude. Remembering to stay in a state of appreciation for each bite of food that we eat allows the feeling of satisfaction to increase. This connects with mindfulness as well; we need to stay in the present moment when we eat and be aware of all the people that brought us this food and all the hands that prepared it or packaged it. Staying in a space of gratitude allows us to be satisfied with what we have, instead of our attention being focused on getting more, more, more. Gratitude will be discussed further in Chapter Five.

What we say or don't say to ourselves while we're eating can be the key to whether or not we stay aware and deliberate in our approach to food. Moment by moment, observe your process and have compassion for yourself.

Write down some examples of your own self-talk to support and empower you when food gets tempting. Some of my own examples are: "I'm capable of meeting my own needs," "I don't need this food right now," "I don't have to keep eating just because my eating companions are still eating." And the most basic: "I don't need food right now...it is my mind talking, not my stomach or my body needing fuel." I don't have to punish myself through food whenever I question if I'm handling my emotions in that moment.

Managing our self-talk by monitoring and interrupting negative thoughts and inserting positive ones is a way to navigate our way to a healthy choice. It is a way to feel empowered.

Exercise 3

Use the space below for your positive self-talk for the next time you are around food.

_____

_____

_____

_____

_____

_____

_____

_____

_____

_____

_____

A *Meditation*:

Breathe in and breathe out; breathe in and breathe out. Take in your surroundings and feel at peace. Feel a feel a sense of calmness and security, knowing that you have what it takes to manage your self- talk, moment by moment. See yourself taking the time to pause and contemplate and to say positive, affirming statements to yourself when you are making choices around food. Know that by remembering to congratulate yourself on your successes, one step at a time, you are building a foundation for further success, enhancing your self-confidence and self-esteem.

CHAPTER FIVE

GRATITUDE

Step 1: Self Awareness

- How can I be more thankful for the food I have?
- How can I remind myself to take smaller portions and be grateful for that amount of food instead of wanting more?
- How can I stay in the present, focusing on each bite that I have, and being grateful for this nourishment?
- How can I remind myself to chew my food completely and fully instead of gulping it down and wanting more before I have even swallowed?

Gratitude is a brilliant tool for managing the quantity and quality of the food we eat. By acknowledging the food that is at our disposal and consuming it gratefully, there is a shift in our approach to food. We don't need as much food to feel full because we are satisfied with less. Our attention is on feeling thankful vs. "this is not enough." The feeling of gratitude fills up our souls, not just our stomachs, and allows us to feel nourished on all levels.

Repeating, "I am grateful for this food," with each bite shifts you into a space of appreciation.

Appreciation quiets your yearning for more.

 When we nourish ourselves with positive self-talk and positive views of the world and our immediate surroundings, we feel better. We feel filled up. We no longer have the sense of an empty void inside us that needs to be numbed and stuffed with food.

Exercise 4

When you eat, focus on being thankful for each small bite. When you chew, chew with appreciation, and really taste the flavor in a way that you have never tasted food before. With each bite, contemplate how grateful you are to be eating and focus on the fact that this food will nourish your body. Have appreciation for all the hands it took to get this food to you, all the way from wherever it grew. Marvel at the long journey this food has been on, and give thanks that it has made it into your hands. You are now thankful that you have food and the means to nourish your body.

Strategies for Nourishing Yourself

Ask yourself: what are some other ways that I can achieve a sense of feeling nourished and fulfilled at this moment?

- Take a bubble bath.
- Reconnect with a friend or family member.

- Spend time with a pet.
- Enjoy a new hobby.
- Light a candle.
- Listen to some music.
- Immerse yourself in a spiritual ritual, such as prayer.
- Seek spiritual support.
- Crawl into bed with a good book.
- Take a walk.
- Go on a hike.
- Smell the roses.
- Water the flowers
- Play a sport.
- Write in a journal.
- Add some of your personal favorites:

_____

_____

_____

A Meditation:

As I take a breath in, I remember that nourishment comes from many different sources. I am nourishing myself with all my senses, not just my stomach. I am feeding myself throughout the day with my eyes, ears, and nose. I am nourishing myself with what I say to myself spiritually and how I view myself and others in the great cosmos. I feed myself by surrounding myself with attractive reminders of natural beauty, those I love, and those who love me. I am grateful for all that I have and for all the lives I touch and for those who touch mine.

CHAPTER SIX

EATING LIGHT AND RIGHT FOR ME

- How much food does my body need during the day?
- How many meals a day work for my schedule and my body's needs?
- What kinds of food give me the most energy during the day?

Successful dieters often remark that much of their success is because they have planned their snacks as well as their meals. They have thought ahead and planned for the awkward, impulsive moments when they want to eat. Having something healthy in front of them avoids the sudden, frantic trips to the vending machines or snack shop.

Readiness to change is also important. People who are not ready to change their behaviors will not be successful because they are unwilling to experience the discomfort that comes with altering a habit that has become part of their automatic behavior. You have to be prepared to stay on top of the behavior, to monitor your thoughts and actions, to pace yourself differently when you are around food. In essence, food needs to become something quite different to you than it was before.

People who are not ready often respond with some variation of the following:

"I have too much going on in my life to focus on eating right."

"I'm under stress; it's not a good time."
"When I take smaller portions and smaller bites, I feel deprived and that makes me feel uncomfortable. I feel like I am starving myself."

"I don't have the patience to plan all of my meals ahead of time." "I've been eating this way my whole lifetime; I can't change now."

"I've tried every diet plan and none of them work." "It's just easier to eat the way I want to. It makes me happy. It's comfort food."

Think about it—if there was nothing in the way, everyone would be at their perfect weight.

So, what is stopping all the people in the world from weighing exactly what they wish? It varies; for everyone it is different. It may be "loving food," not wanting to feel deprived, using food to handle emotions or cope with stress, physiology, hating to exercise or a slower metabolism (which happens to everyone as we get older.) Add to this the time spent commuting or in front of computers, and you see a sedentary nation now used to supersized portions.

Remember the basic principle that you must burn more calories than you eat in order to lose weight. In other words, the energy that goes out (is burned off) must be more than the energy you take in (food); you have to either take in fewer calories or exercise more to lose weight.

Each of us must decide what we will change and then turn our attention to re-creating ourselves. Here is an opportunity to specify the new habits and routines you will practice to live the way you imagine yourself to be.

Here are some examples:

- Get up earlier a few days a week to exercise.
- Spend your lunch hour walking.
- Walk before or after dinner.
- Resist dessert, except for special occasions.
- Choose healthier snack alternatives at work or school: carrots, celery, or fruit for example.
- Avoid food after _ pm.
- Stand up and move around at least once an hour.

Exercise 5

It is important to keep a food journal, to help you monitor every morsel of food you put into your mouth. After writing in your food journal when you are about to eat, see if you can see the patterns emerging. Do you notice you eat more at different times of the day, such as 4 pm? Do you eat more when you are stressed? Do you eat more when you feel that things are out of control, and you feel you don't have the answer? Record the themes you have noticed:

- I eat a lot when (ex: I am experiencing stress)

_____

_____

_____

- I tend to snack when (ex.: I get home from work and am tired)

  _____

  _____

  _____

- I find myself overeating when (ex: I feel out of control with work demands)

  _____

  _____

  _____

- I notice that I turn to food I know is not good for me when (ex. I am overtired) _____

  and then I feel _____ afterwards.

Then after you have been practicing your new habits, you can see new patterns such as: "when I kept reminding myself one portion was enough," or "when I was able to say no to sugar because it gives me a headache," or "when I told myself to stop snacking because it wouldn't help me reach my goal any faster."

- I I was successful in avoiding extra portions when

  _____

  _____

  _____

- was able to stop snacking when I told myself

_____

_____

_____

- I used this trick to avoid mindless eating

_____

_____

_____

- At four in the afternoon when the afternoon slump hit, I tried a new habit of

_____

_____

_____

- At eight at night when I thought I was hungry, I

_____

_____

_____

- When my friends and family were gobbling away, I tried a new routine of

_____

_____

_____

Keep track of your positive phrases. These are the phrases that keep you fulfilled and the words that give you energy. List them here or in your food journal.

Words and phrases that nourish me:

I have had enough food. Stop!
Pause
Breathe
I am enough without this food
It's possible
I can do this
It's easy for me to eat less food than I used to
because I now care for my body

Some of your own important words and phrases:

_____

_____

_____

_____

_____

_____

_____

_____

A Meditation:

Take a deep breath and as you breathe in and out, in and out, imagine a sense of peace and calm coming over your body. As you continue to take nice easy breaths, start to see yourself practicing these small but meaningful steps, one by one. See yourself being able to make these deliberate choices each day, which all add up to major changes in your lifestyle. Observe yourself saying no to excess food, saying no to eating mindlessly, or triumphing over whatever has been challenging you. Notice that with each challenge you successfully navigate, you feel stronger and more confident, allowing yourself to meet the next challenge with ease and certainty. It is becoming easier and easier to eat the way you prefer—making healthy choices. As you come back to waking space, you bring with you.

CHAPTER SEVEN

NOW WHAT: YOUR NEW EATING
BLUEPRINT STARTS NOW

Practice keeping your long-term vision and goal of a brand-new, conscious self by writing goals in your food journal and noticing your self-talk. Write down what your thoughts are and what you say to yourself when you are around food. Pay attention to what you are feeling before you eat and eat mindfully and slowly. Eventually you won't need to consciously ask yourself, "Why am I eating this?" any longer because mindfulness will have become a part of who you are. You will have successfully reconditioned and retrained yourself in a powerful, positive way. You will have naturally heightened your awareness around food, and you will be able to make choices that reflect a happy, healthy vision of you.

The key is to continue using your awareness and intention every time you are around food. Use your newfound wisdom to eat consciously and deliberately. Stay in touch with your emotions/feelings, your actions, and your thoughts at all times. Remind yourself to assess your level of hunger, i.e., "how hungry am I right now"? before you eat.

By following the steps outlined in this book : paying attention, eating mindfully, remembering your eating history, using positive self-talk, having gratitude, and eating light and right for your fuel needs, you have in fact been re-designing your personal eating blue-print.

YOU CAN DESIGN YOUR EATING BLUEPRINT!

Example:

I always have some protein at every meal.
I keep my blood sugar stable by eating every 3 hours.

I always carry healthy snacks with me, so I am not caught in between meals craving unhealthy snacks.

Exercise is an important part of my life: a minimum of 30 minutes every day.

I stay aware of how hungry I am and stop eating before I feel full.

In social situations, I use positive self-talk to stay aware and not overeat because of emotions or because everyone else is stuffing themselves.

MY EATING BLUEPRINT

_____

_____

_____

_____

_____

_____

_____

_____

THIS NEW WAY OF EATING WILL BE A PART OF WHO YOU ARE

I have heard people say, "Dieting is a mind game." It is really true. There are many ways to play the game and many strategies developed by countless experts and weight-loss gurus. But in the end, it is a choice between you and the food, between you and your mind, each and every time you are around food. What is it that you say to yourself? Do your words nourish or defeat you?

It is my prayer that after reading this book, you will have new and exciting strategies linking you and your mind to success. You will have new tools and strategies to change your approach to food, for a lifetime. You will be reminded to pause when you are around food, and you feel that old temptation to eat "just because." Turn your attention to making good, healthy choices by monitoring your thoughts, emotions, and behavior your thoughts, emotions, and behavior and developing self-talk that supports and nourishes you.

This powerful combination: attention, seeing the link between your thoughts, emotions and behavior, and positive self-talk will be the keys to a new you whenever you are around food.

To your good health and success!

A Meditation:

Take a deep breath in and let it go; take another breath in, breathing nourishment from the universe into your lungs. You are aware that you are bringing vital energy into your body. As you take another deep breath in, see yourself taking care of your body in a new, healthy way. As you continue to take nice easy breaths, imagine yourself living in a new way. See yourself taking in only the food you need and being aware of when you are eating for reasons other than bodily nourishment. Breathing in life, breathing out fear or distress, you feel a calm sense of certainty that you have what it takes to accomplish your goal. See yourself letting go of lifelong patterns that did not serve you, and instead, inserting new ones with your newfound knowledge and the awareness that you can talk to yourself in new, healthy, and supporting ways when you are around food. See yourself making positive changes, day by day, taking only as much as you need, and it becomes easier and easier to make these wise and deliberate choices. As you embrace this vision, you see the result in front of you: a healthy new you at your perfect new weight.

CHAPTER EIGHT

AN ADDENDUM

Since I published *Why Am I Eating This?* in 2009, many people have told me that it helped them rethink how they view food and modify many of their eating habits. They have shared that they now pay attention to their eating speed and, as a result, eat slower. Many have also reported paying more attention to the bags of sweet or crispy treats that help them get through a rough day at work but don't provide any helpful fuel for their bodies. Some notice that they were eating based on emotions "just like their mother" and are now tuning in to how they feel before they grab a snack "just because."

In the many hours spent teaching mindful eating, mind-body-stress hardiness, and counseling people on adopting healthier eating patterns, the one theme that keeps reappearing is that people often grab food without a thought of whether it is nourishing or good for their bodies. They wonder why they are tired, can't sleep, have digestive challenges, or can't think straight, and they don't stop to think if it might have something to do with the quality of fuel that they are putting into their bodies. The other theme I have heard is, "I eat healthy food, but way too much of it." These clients say they eat healthy food, but their portion sizes are too large. Selecting the "right" nourishment also involves selecting the right amount!

This 2nd edition of my book offers some fine-tuning on the concept of choosing food as nourishment. It pushes the reader to look with intention at areas where they can find other sources of nourishment in their lives. This new, enriched version takes the original 7 steps found in my book *Why Am I Eating This?* and adds 7 more steps around the theme of "nourishment."

The question this book digs deeper into is:

- "Will this nourish my body . . . and my soul?"
- "How else can I nourish my body, mind, spirit, and energy system?"

THE SEVEN NEW QUESTIONS

1. **Am I seeking "fuel" (calories) instead of self-care?**

Sometimes I notice when I reach for a snack that I'm feeling an emotion that's uncomfortable, and I am seeking comfort. Even if it is annoyance with a tech issue that feels impossible in the moment ... a deep breath, an "oh well, I can figure this out or call tech support to hear a kind, helpful voice" may be the kind of nourishment I need. Or, if I'm tired and want to eat, I remind myself, "I'm tired, not hungry." At other times, I pause and remember that 5 minutes of breathing, lighting a candle, or a quick call to a friend might help shift the feeling of "I want to eat." Perhaps instead, it is "I want connection" or "I need support with this issue I'm trying to resolve." See if you can list 5 non-food ways to practice self-care that work for you.

Nutrition as "Fuel": How would it be to think of what we put in our mouths as "fuel"? As nutrients for our body, with vitamins, minerals, and helpful micro-elements for our body and *brain* (see Chapter 9 - "Neuro Nutrition")?

The original version of *Why Am I Eating This?* specifically addressed rethinking how you view food in three chapters: **Self-Talk, Eating Light and Right for Me and Discover Your Food Patterns.** I want to add to the concept of thinking of food as "fuel" in more depth. Many friends and clients mention, "I can't lose weight." There are various reasons for the inability to lose weight, which may depend on the person and their unique metabolic composition. One basic reason for holding onto weight is not enough exercise or energy expenditure compared to the "energy" or calories taken in. (Once again, discuss your unique metabolic issues with a doctor or dietician.)

But many clients who are successful at losing weight are willing to start viewing food as "fuel." So that a majority of the time, they are willing to ask themselves, "Is this the best fuel for my body right now?" Do I need protein for energy and brain fuel instead of a cup of coffee? Or would a complex carbohydrate like fruit be good instead of empty calories in chips, crackers, pretzels, etc.? (These are foods that I love—I just have to be deliberate when I eat them!)

And if you look at it from the perspective that you have a certain "fuel allotment" for the day, depending on your age and other demographic statistics, then you know generally you have approximately 1400 (women) or 1800 (men) calories to "spend" throughout the day. (These are very general numbers. Please always consult your doctor or dietician for more specific guidance.) For example: "If I have 1400 calories available to me for the day, do I really want to eat 700 calories worth of chocolate or chips right now?"

Looking at "food as fuel" is the ultimate form of self-love—it is caring for yourself enough to care about what you ingest. It is wanting to put the highest quality food and drink into your body most of the time. Thinking about "food as fuel" will then help pose other questions . . . **How much is enough?** Even good "fuel" such as proteins, fruits, and whole grains can be too much.

When is it wise to say "stop"? Can I be satisfied with less if I chew more, breaking my food into smaller parts, which eases digestion? Can I reduce my portion size, slow down my eating (extending the length of time I eat), and not feel deprived? These are great questions when you are willing to ponder the meaning of food in your life in deeper ways as a form of nourishment. Considering "How much is enough" will allow you to self-nurture in new ways!

2. **How would I label these calories (from a place of non-judgment)?**

Am I about to choose "empty" calories with not much nutritional value? Where is the nourishment? How will I feel when I eat this? How will it affect me physically and psychologically? Will it elevate my mood? Give me more energy? Satisfy a craving . . . but then be a source of shame, anger, or regret?

"Studies in recent years suggest that the sugar-laden and high-fat foods we often crave when we are stressed or depressed . . . are the least likely to benefit our mental health."[1] How would we feel about including more whole foods, proteins, grains, legumes, fruits, and vegetables, adjusted to whatever diet we follow for health, spiritual/religious reasons, or both? Ask yourself some of these questions:

- **Do I really want to put this in my grocery cart?** Dieticians and nutritionists speak of shopping the perimeter of a grocery store to fill your cart with fruits, vegetables, nuts, and proteins of your choosing. Nutrition expert Ashley Cornell, BASc, Applied Human Nutrition Bariatric Educator, shares: "Shop the produce section first. If you load up your basket with fresh fruits and vegetables, you are less likely to succumb to the urge to put additional snack foods in your basket."[2] A study done by Civic Science, a market research group, interviewed shoppers who said they buy fresh foods.

---

[1] O'Connor, A. (2021, May 6). How food may improve your mood. The New York Times. Retrieved May 2, 2023, from https://www.nytimes.com/2021/05/06/well/eat/mental-health-food.html
[2] Cornell, Ashley. Wharton Medical Clinic. Accessed May 12, 2023. https://whartonmedicalclinic.com/handouts/Perimeter%20Shopping.pdf.

But when more specific questions were asked, they were actually buying mostly packaged and prepared foods. "The group surveyed about 5800 adults and found that in the past year, only 20 percent of those surveyed spent 50 percent of their total supermarket budget on fresh foods."[3]

- **"Is this something to entertain me . . . or nourish me?** If it's entertainment, that's great; just label it that way so you start to become aware of how often you are seeking entertainment via food. Could you add other forms of entertainment to your life? Or, if you admit that "Yes, in fact, this is pure entertainment," then go ahead and ENJOY!! Have fun!!!! But . . . could you still have fun with something somewhat healthy? Or could you limit the number of times each week that you are turning to food for entertainment . . . perhaps on weekends, for example?

A great article on this topic is "Obesity a Malnourished State - Real Food is the Answer" by Roxanne B. Sukol.[4] As she so eloquently states, "Real Food comes from 11 categories ..." She then describes things like protein sources/fruits and vegetables, beans, whole grains, nuts, and seeds. Things that nature produces! She goes on to state: "That is food. Everything else is fun, which entertains but does not nourish."

---

[3] Hendel, Amy. A smart diet: Shop the market perimeter to be healthy. Accessed May 12, 2023. https://www.healthcentral. com/article/a-smart-diet-shop-the-market-perimeter-to-be-healthy.

[4] Sukol, R. B. (2019). Obesity A Malnourished State - Real Food is the Answer. Alternative and Complementary Medicine, 25(5). https://doi. org/10.1089/acm.2019.29020.rbs

3. **Will this serve my gut? The brain and the stomach are linked!**

Have you heard of the "gut-brain connection"? Even if you are not a scientist or dietician, you may have noticed that what you eat affects your mood and how you feel. Consequently, if you feel low or depressed, you are drawn to unhealthy foods that taste great and are comforting. But high-calorie/low-nutrient foods aren't necessarily good for you and can alter the quality of bacteria in your gut. (And there are "good" bacteria in our gut, which help many processes in the body.) Also, according to researchers Annelise Madison and Janice K Kiecolt-Glaser[1] in their article "Stress, depression, diet, and the gut microbiota: human bacteria interactions at the core of psychoneuroimmunology and nutrition," stress and depression can alter the gut bacteria's composition.

They discuss how gut bacteria may release toxins and other elements that can change our eating behavior and mood in response to stress and hormonal changes.

Another resource comes from the National Institute of Health Division of Complementary/ Integrative Health:

[1] Madison, A., Kiecolt-Glaser, J. K. Stress, depression, diet, and the gut microbiota: human-bacteria interactions at the core of psychoneuroimmunology and nutrition. Curr Opin Behav Sci. 2019 Aug; 28:105-110. doi: 10.1016/j.cobeha.2019.01.011. Epub 2019 Mar 25. PMID: 32395568; PMCID: PMC7213601.

"4 Fast Facts About the Gut-Brain Connection"

1. "Gut Microbiota" are bacteria that live in your intestine.
2. The gut and the brain communicate in two different ways: the brain communicates with the gut, as when you have a "gut reaction."
3. The gut microbiota can go in the other direction and affect the brain. Probiotic bacteria can help calm anxiety, according to Dr. Cryan (2011) (NIH/NCCIH)
4. Altering the diet by altering bacteria in the gut may help stress-related illnesses.
   Source: www.nccih.nih.gov[6]

Scores of articles and research are now being done on the "gut-brain connection," and the term "brain in your gut" is now being used more to describe the intricate inter-workings of all of the bacteria and neurotransmitters in your stomach that communicate with your brain, and affect your mood, health, and emotions, digestion, and more.

"Neuro-Nutrition" is an emerging field studying the effects of certain nutrients on the functions of the brain and cognitive health. There are even college courses on Neuro-Nutrition, several books, and countless supplements promising the magic bullet for "Neuro-Nutrition."

Of course, food supplies energy to our bodies, but it is now reminding us that it has the capacity for medicinal purposes, improving molecular processes, which can improve mental function.

_____

6   "NCCIH." National Center for Complementary and Integrative Health. Accessed May 12, 2023. http://www.nccih.nih.gov/.

Scientists are now linking food and the brain, including research on specific diets that can slow the symptoms of certain diseases. Nutrients also can affect neurotransmitters, the chemical messengers in the body. They are part of the nervous system, which impacts almost all bodily functions. Serotonin, the neurotransmitter that lets our brain know we are relaxed, also affects sleep and appetite regulation. Many people have heard of the "runner's high" and the release of serotonin. Few people know that *food* contributes to the creation of serotonin and that the amino acid tryptophan (found in many foods, including, yes, turkey) contributes to serotonin production (90% of serotonin is actually produced in the intestines).

Foods rich in tryptophan include chia seeds, whole milk, sesame seeds, plain whole-milk yogurt, pumpkin seeds (a source of omega-3 fatty acids and vitamin E), prunes, seaweed, spirulina, raw cacao, whole-grain wheat bread (which also contains vitamin E), and edamame. Fermented foods have also gotten a lot of press lately for having the potential to improve brain and cognitive function. There is research suggesting that eating fermented food can influence the central nervous system. The premise is that fermentation helps to break down food and shift the chemical composition of food, making the food more "bioavailable." It may also help with intestinal absorption of nutrients in the body. Furthermore, research is showing that probiotics in fermented food may shift gut microorganisms and influence brain function via the gut-brain connection.[7]

[7] Kim, B., Hong, V. M., Yang, J., Hyun, H., Im, J. J., Hwang, J., Yoon, S., & Kim, J. E. (2016, December). A review of fermented foods with beneficial effects on brain and cognitive function.
Preventive nutrition and food science. Retrieved May 2, 2023, from https://www.ncbi.nlm.nih.gov/pmc/articles/PMC5216880/

Medical News Today published an online article titled "12 foods to boost brain function."[8] These top foods are as follows: **oily fish** (a good source of omega-3 fatty acids), **dark chocolate** (a good source of flavonoids, an antioxidant), **berries** (another good source of flavonoids), **nuts and seeds, whole grains, coffee** (shown to help with focus), **avocados** (a healthful source of unsaturated fat), **peanuts** (an unsaturated fat), **eggs** (a good source of vitamin B6, vitamin B12, and folic acid), **broccoli** (a great cruciferous vegetable with lots of fiber and other healthy vitamins), **kale** (contains glucosinolates and other healthy vitamins, good for brain health), and **soy** (contains isoflavones, which are antioxidants).

In summary, the emerging field of "neuro-nutrition" involves adding some new "why am I eating this" questions to check in about the value of this food for your brain health!

Many of the suggestions mirror other recommended diets; as always, check in with your health care provider about a specific diet for your medical needs. But in general, the guidance of neuro-nutrition includes antioxidant-rich foods, such as dark leafy greens, nuts, seeds, and berries; omega-3 fatty acids (found in fatty fish, flaxseeds, chia seeds, and walnuts); staying hydrated (helpful for brain function since dehydration can impair brain function); limiting processed foods and added sugars (may contribute to inflammation in the body, which can affect brain health). In addition, eating mindfully (a theme of this book) is frequently a recommendation from doctors and dieticians.

---

8   Burgess, L. (n.d.). 12 best brain foods: Memory, concentration, and Brain Health. Medical News Today. https://www.medicalnewstoday.com/articles/324044

Slowing down the eating/snacking process can help create new habits around intentional eating . . . because you are practicing self-care!

4. **Timing is everything!**

When did I last eat? What food patterns and food rhythms are right for me? Some people find it helpful to eat every few hours instead of skipping meals or having long stretches in between meals. When your blood sugar drops, it can cause you to feel HANGRY (feeling angry, but you are really hungry!). Here is another mnemonic to think about before you go for a snack: "HALT" – are you Hungry, Angry, Lonely, or

Hungry
Angry
Lonely
Tired ?

Tired? Once you have taken the time to reflect, you have time to choose again!!

Planning meals and snacks in advance can help you to have a sense of control over your intake and know you will have the healthy foods/meals that nourish you all lined up. If you are eating out, having a sense of the choices you will make before you get there may help too.

There are many food trends now around practicing "time-based eating" and intermittent fasting is one of them.

Intermittent fasting involves avoiding food for a certain number of hours to give the body's digestive system a rest and reset metabolism. This process has shown that it may benefit your weight, heart, mind, and overall health. The three most popular types of intermittent fasting strategies are outlined in the UCLA Health article "Health benefits of intermittent fasting (and tips for making it work)"[9]:

- **Alternate Day Fasting:** Normal eating every other day, with days of restricted eating (500 calories) in between.

- **Daily time-restricted eating:** Limits the window when you can eat each day (usually six to eight hours). The rest of the time, you are fasting.

- **5:2 approach:** Normal eating five days a week, but restricting calories to 500-600 calories/day, two days a week, not in a row).

Intermittent fasting can work because when your body is deprived of food for several hours, it runs out of the usual source of energy (recently eaten food stored as sugar) and starts burning fat. During intermittent fasting, the body instead turns to fat to produce energy. This is why people lose weight, can improve their diabetes and insulin sensitivity, and gain other health benefits. (Be sure to discuss this with your physician before starting any kind of fasting program.)

---

[9] Health benefits of intermittent fasting (and tips for making it work). UCLA Health System. (n.d.). Retrieved May 2, 2023, from https://www.uclahealth.org/news/health-benefits-of-intermittent-fasting-and-tips-for-making-it-work

5. **What else nourishes me? What other kinds of nourishment am I seeking?**

What would it be like to think of what we put in our mouths as nourishment that will have an impact on our souls, not just our bodies? In his book *The Hungry Soul*,[10] Dr. Leonard Kass, MD, writes about the "relationship between what one is and what one eats." He says, "Eating comes to satisfy appetites for more than nutrition, and not only among human beings."

Consider what nourishes you. Is it nature, friends, music, art, aromas, or social or spiritual gatherings? Many health coaches use a "circle of health," also known as a "wheel of health," with many of these elements of healthy living artfully arranged in a circle to assess which areas need more support. It is a visual reminder that to be at optimum wellness, our minds, bodies, spirits, and energy systems need to be in sync and attended to. Just for a moment, ask yourself, "How am I doing on sleep? On social support? On spiritual nourishment? And overall, on things that bring me joy?"

Take a moment to recall when you feel nourished . . . other than with food. Where are you? Who are you with or talking to? What are your surroundings like? From that point of view, ask yourself, "How much nourishment do I need in each area?" Or "Why do I sometimes over-nourish my body with food?"

---

10   Kass, L. R. (1999). The hungry soul: Eating and the perfecting of our nature. The University of Chicago Press.

Ask these questions not from a place of blame or judgment but as a neutral observer. Like a friend, gently ask yourself: Is there something else I need? Another kind of nourishment that's not food? How about sleep?

The power of sleep is often forgotten. Recent research has shown that inadequate sleep can result in various health challenges, including obesity and hormonal imbalances. Changes in our circadian rhythm can upset our blood sugar and insulin balance, resulting in increased cravings for caffeine, junk food, and sugary snacks to compensate for the lack of energy. These habits can put individuals at a higher risk of developing diabetes.[11,12]

---

11 Lazar, M. A., & Adlanmerini, M. (2021). A 'Dented' Internal Clock Provides Insight Into Shift Workers' Weight Gain and Diabetes. Science Advances, 7(44), eabm1239. https://doi.org/10.1126/sciadv.abm1239

12 Lazar, M. A., & Adlanmerini, M. (2021, October 28). A 'Dented' Internal Clock Provides Insight Into Shift Workers' Weight Gain and Diabetes. Penn Medicine News. https://www.pennmedicine.org/news/news-releases/2021/october/dented-internal-clock-provides-insight-into-shift-workers-weight-gain-and-diabetes

6. **Self-care is self-nourishment (Nourishment comes in many forms.)**

In my work as a mind/body/spirit/energy system coach, I invite my clients to tune into these four areas of their lives for a quick check-in.

Mind - Positive self-talk is a form of self-love. Take a minute to consider your thoughts and the quality of your "self-talk" throughout the day. Are you saying life-affirming, uplifting statements to yourself? Or are you sabotaging your goals and dreams by saying, "I'm afraid . . . I can't do it . . . what if I re-injure myself . . . what if I fail? I invite my clients to say self-affirming statements to themselves. I often refer clients to Louise Hay's book *You Can Heal Your Life*[13] for simple, positive statements.

Body - How much are you moving your body, getting up and moving around during the day, stretching, and breathing, in addition to more formal kinds of classes or exercise?

---

13 Hay, L. L. (2017). You can heal your life. Hay House, Inc.

Some people say they don't have time to "exercise," but the reality is that they could incorporate more movement into everyday rhythms. Getting up once an hour and moving around, parking farther away in the parking garage, or taking the stairs instead of an escalator or elevator. Taking 20-minute walks twice a day. These are all great ways to incorporate "movement." Breathing techniques can help you to refresh and restart the moment and help you to choose food and amounts from a deliberate, grounded place.

How about sleep? As mentioned above, if we are sleep deprived, we frequently crave sugar and carbohydrates, or "fast calories." Our circadian rhythms are thrown off, causing our chemical messenger system and hormones to seek calories that will give us quick energy. Research has shown that people who work the night shift frequently gain weight because our bodies are programmed to eat when it's light, not when it's dark.[14] Achieving a natural sleep pattern will improve your overall health. Chronic Stress can also impact sleep patterns, which in turn can affect your energy and mental clarity in the following days. Focusing on "Sleep Hygiene" (steps to cue your body and the environment to ensure restful, peaceful sleep) can improve health and contribute to a rested, relaxed, and healthy body.

Many of us carry around a water bottle, but then forget to take sips throughout the day. Dehydration can contribute to feeling tired, as well as affect other aspects of our health. We may feel like we want to take a nap when what we really need is some water!

------

[14] University of Colorado Boulder, 2014, November 17. Working the night shift burns less energy and increases risk of weight gain. https://www.colorado.edu/today/2014/11/17/working-night-shift-burns-less-energy-and-increases-risk-weight-gain

Spirit - Do you have a connection with a higher power or spirit; however, you define that? Do you feel supported by God/your highest wisdom/the Universe in a way that helps you make sense of the world around you and your place in it? Albert Einstein is quoted as saying, "I think the most important question facing humanity is 'Is the universe a friendly place?'" Having a source of spiritual support and feeling good about your place in the world can help you feel supported.

Turning to spiritual support can help you feel connected to the earth and others, so you do not feel alone. And social support among like-minded people can help too. Some have found Overeaters Anonymous (OA) and other support groups to be very helpful with coaching support and a group that truly understands your cravings and issues around food.

Energy System - Our bodies are made up of energy . . . we are an energy system. Through the centuries, this has been referred to as chi, qi, prana, and many other names. Our energy systems are affected by our body mechanisms, but also our thoughts and emotions. (i.e., thoughts of fear can affect the sympathetic nervous system). We are also affected by the energy outside of us . . . in the environment, technology, and even crowded spaces. Have you ever gone into a room where people have had an argument or are very upset? You can feel the energy is off. Compare this to when you go into a very clear space, with lots of light, plants, nice aromas, and happy people—the energy just feels different . . . lighter! Keep your environment and energy system clear by minimizing the electronics and sometimes the number of people around you.

Keeping a daily self-care journal, where you are also tracking your energy system throughout the day, in addition to checking in on your mind, body, emotions, spirit, self-care habits, and well-being, can help you to get a sense of what brings you joy and fosters good habits versus the situations or people that create more stress . . . and are a trigger for you to overeat.

7. How about a dose of self-compassion instead of a sugary snack?

A growing body of research on the helpfulness of self-compassion (the ability to give oneself loving kindness, tenderness, and comfort during times of distress) shows that-self compassion may also be helpful for people trying to lose weight or practice healthy lifestyle habits. One systematic review (a review of many research articles) evaluated studies that looked at self-compassion and weight management; of the 9082 research records screened, 17 studies reported "significant increases in self-compassion post-intervention. Improvements were also found for eating behaviors, physical activity behaviors, and weight loss."[15]

In her article "Self-compassion: An alternate conceptualization of a healthy attitude toward oneself," Dr. Kristin Neff, Ph.D., describes how self-compassion consists of self-kindness, common humanity, and mindfulness.[16]

In a separate research study, Drs. Michail Mantzios and Helen H. Egan looked at some explanations as to why and how self-compassion can help people who wish to change their eating

---

[15] Brenton-Peters, J., et al. (2021, November). J Psychosom Res.

[16] Neff, K. D. (2003). Self-compassion: An alternate conceptualization of a healthy attitude toward oneself. Self and Identity, 2(2), 85-101. https://doi.org/10.1080/15298860309032

patterns. Among other elements of the study, participants kept an "event-based diary/exercise to be used with every meal and aimed at increasing mindfulness and self-compassionate levels when eating."[17] The article discussed how mindful self-compassion during eating introduced themes of mindfulness and intuitive eating. All of this awareness in the present moment helped people be more deliberate.

The premise of offering oneself self-compassion when eating is that if we tend to "eat our emotions"—with eating sometimes serving as a way to numb our feelings—then if we offer ourselves a loving, healthy alternative in the form of attending to our emotional needs when eating, with present-minded awareness and care, we will be more deliberate with our food choices and amounts because our emotions are being simultaneously attended to. In other words, instead of "stuffing our feelings," we can offer ourselves loving kindness when eating.

Of course, we are hurting. Of course, we are sad or angry. But still, we can decide to put the right amount of healthy nourishment into our bodies in a loving way.

Self-compassion research and training often include "loving kindness" phrases (originated with a form of mediation), which are statements to the self to call forth self-soothing and comfort.

---

[17] Mantzios, M., & Egan, H. H. (2017). On the role of self-compassion and self-kindness in weight regulation and health behavior change. Frontiers in Psychology, 8, 229. https://doi.org/10.3389/fpsyg.2017.00229

Examples may include:

May I be happy?
May I be peaceful?
May I be joyful?
May I be courageous?
May I trust in the present moment?

CONCLUSION

Why Am I Eating This . . . Is this the nourishment I need? is a call to the self-love we all want to give ourselves and deserve. Start practicing some of these simple techniques while formulating new, simple, and fun ways to honor, respect, and care for yourself. Turn to all the professional resources you need (therapy, counseling, doctor and dietician, 12-step programs) to support you in deepening your path of self-love.

EPILOGUE

I have been writing this book for seven years. It has gone through many edits and revisions. It has been waiting for one final piece.

"Our outer actions are a reflection of our inner feelings about ourselves." (Author unknown.)

Unless we feel good about ourselves inside, we will not take the steps to care for our outer package, our body that is a gift from God.

Outer self-care reflects inner self love and appreciation.

When we love and cherish ourselves, we will want to love and cherish our bodies and will not want to continually overfill it with fuel that is not good for us.

Keep your thoughts and self-talk positive and filled with self-love. Then your actions will reflect your positive self-image.

Your love and appreciation for yourself will be reflected in good care, good habits, and good health.

If you need help shifting your thoughts to ones that are positive about yourself, seek the assistance of a qualified psychologist or psychotherapist. You may benefit from working with a professional mental health expert who can guide you through past inner traumas or painful wounds that are affecting how you feel about yourself today. Consider it just a normal part of a "self-care package" to get the professional guidance that can help you understand why you might be sabotaging yourself with overeating. An expert mental health professional can help you release the past, get to the bottom of why you are overeating for emotional reasons, and give you tools to focus on the present.

We all need help and guidance to understand ourselves and what is at the root of our habits and patterns. Give yourself the gift of discovering what is in your emotional history that can give you insight and ultimately the freedom to start anew.

As part of this newfound freedom, you can create healthy habits and patterns that are based on the present and not the past.

This book is not meant to take the place of therapy, it is merely intended to provide clues to the puzzle, "Why am I eating this?"

The real message here is that you don't have to be on this journey alone. There are also meditation classes, spiritual support, psychotherapy, and books that can guide and support you in this process.

Surround yourself with people who reflect back to you all of your beauty and goodness and remind you of all of your positive qualities. Your willingness to take a look at your habits and thoughts will start you on a path of awareness that will shift how you approach food. You will never look at food the same way again.... well, you might look, but your thoughts will turn to "Why Am I Eating This"?

Have fun with this new approach to food and let me know how you are doing.

I wish you luck, but most of all success and triumph over food.

Your love and appreciation for yourself will result in good self-care, good habits and good health.

Know that you are worth it. You can envision and create your best self and have all of your self-care and self-nourishment habits reflect the beauty of the real you.

I know you will succeed.

BIBLIOGRAPHY

Burns, David. 1980. *Feeling Good: The New Mood Therapy*. New York: Harper Collins. Revised and updated, 1999. Preface by Aaron T. Beck, MD.

"Fitness, Diet and Body Type." *WorldFitness.org*, 2007. www.worldfitness.org/fitness_body_type.html.

Kabat-Zinn, Jon, 1990, "Full Catastrophe Living", Random House.

Kabat-Zinn, Jon. 1994. *Wherever You Go, There You Are*. New York: Hyperion.

Kristeller, Jean. 2005. "Mindful Eating Research Phase I: Interview with Jean Kristeller, PhD." By Richard Mahler. *eMindful: Interactive Online Courses*, www.emindful.com/interviews/Jean_Kristeller.html.

Lester, Greg. 2005. "Cognitive Therapy Works as well as Antidepressants, but With Lasting Effect after Therapy Ends." Office of University Communications, University of Pennsylvania. http://www.upenn.edu/pennnews/article. php?id=777. April 4, 2005.

Naparstek, Belleruth, 1995, "Staying Well with Guided Imagery", Harper Collins.

Ornstein, Robert and Sobel, David, 1989, "Healthy Pleasures", Addison Wesley.

Ornstein, Robert and Sobel, David, 1998, *The Healthy Mind/ Healthy Body Handbook*, Time Life Books.

Quillian-Wolever, Ruth. 2007. "Mindful Eating Research Phase II & III: Interview with Dr. Ruth Quillian-Wolever, PhD." By Kelly McCabe. *eMindful: Live Interactive Online Courses*, www. emindful.com/interviews/Jean Kristeller.html.

Seligman, Martin. 1990. *Learned Optimism*. New York: Random House.

Tanneeru, Manay. 2006. "Obesity: A looming National Threat," www. cnn.com/2006/Health/diet/fitness. March 24, 2006 (article now discontinued).

Chapter 8 References

Brenton-Peters, J., et al. (2021, November). J Psychosom Res.

Burgess, L. (n.d.). *12 best brain foods: Memory, concentration, and Brain Health*. Medical News Today. https://www. medicalnewstoday.com/articles/324044

Cornell, Ashley. Wharton Medical Clinic. Accessed May 12, 2023. https://whartonmedicalclinic.com/handouts/ Perimeter%20Shopping.pdf.

Complementary Medicine, 25(5). https://doi.org/10.1089/ acm.2019.29020.rbs

Hendel, Amy. A smart diet: Shop the market perimeter to be healthy. Accessed May 12, 2023. https://www.healthcentral.

com/article/a-smart-diet-shop-the-market-perimeter-to-be-healthy.

Hay, L. L. (2017). *You can heal your life*. Hay House, Inc.

Health benefits of intermittent fasting (and tips for making it work). UCLA Health System. (n.d.). Retrieved May 2, 2023, from https://www.uclahealth.org/news/health-benefits-of-intermittent-fasting-and-tips-for-making-it-work

Kass, L. R. (1999). *The hungry soul: Eating and the perfecting of our nature*. The University of Chicago Press.

Kim, B., Hong, V. M., Yang, J., Hyun, H., Im, J. J., Hwang, J., Yoon, S., & Kim, J. E. (2016, December). *A review of fermented foods with beneficial effects on brain and cognitive function*. Preventive nutrition and food science. Retrieved May 2, 2023, from https://www.ncbi.nlm.nih.gov/pmc/articles/PMC5216880/

Lazar, M. A., & Adlanmerini, M. (2021). *A 'Dented' Internal Clock Provides Insight Into Shift Workers' Weight Gain and Diabetes*. Science Advances, 7(44), eabm1239. https://doi.org/10.1126/sciadv.abm1239

Lazar, M. A., & Adlanmerini, M. (2021, October 28). *A 'Dented' Internal Clock Provides Insight Into Shift Workers' Weight Gain and Diabetes*. Penn Medicine News. https://www.pennmedicine.org/news/news-releases/2021/ctober/dented-internal-clock-provides-insight-into-shift-workers-weight-gain-and-diabetes

Madison, A., Kiecolt-Glaser, J. K. *Stress, depression, diet, and the gut microbiota: human-bacteria interactions at the core of psychoneuroimmunology and nutrition*. Curr Opin Behav Sci. 2019 Aug;28:105-110. Doi: 10.1016/j.cobeha.2019.01.011. Epub 2019 Mar 25. PMID: 32395568; PMCID: PMC7213601.

Mantzios, M., & Egan, H. H. (2017). *On the role of self-compassion and self-kindness in weight regulation and health behavior change.* Frontiers in Psychology, 8, 229. https://doi.org/10.3389/fpsyg.2017.00229

"NCCIH." National Center for Complementary and Integrative Health. Accessed May 12, 2023. http://www.nccih.nih.gov/.

Neff, K. D. (2003). *Self-compassion: An alternate conceptualization of a healthy attitude toward oneself.* Self and Identity, 2(2), 85-101. https://doi.org/10.1080/15298860309032

O'Connor, A. (2021, May 6). *How food may improve your mood.* The New York Times. Retrieved May 2, 2023, from https://www.nytimes.com/2021/05/06/well/eat/mental-health-food.html

Sukol, R. B. (2019). *Obesity: A Malnourished State—Real Food Is the Answer.* Alternative and Complementary Therapies, 25(5), 234-237. http://doi.org/10.1089/act.2019.29235.rbs

University of Colorado Boulder, 2014, November 17. *Working the night shift burns less energy and increases risk of weight gain.* https://www.colorado.edu/today/2014/11/17/working-night-shift-burns-less-energy-and-increases-risk-weight-gain

Made in the USA
Las Vegas, NV
27 February 2024

86333781R00056